LIFESTYLE FACTORS AFFECTING CANCER RISK

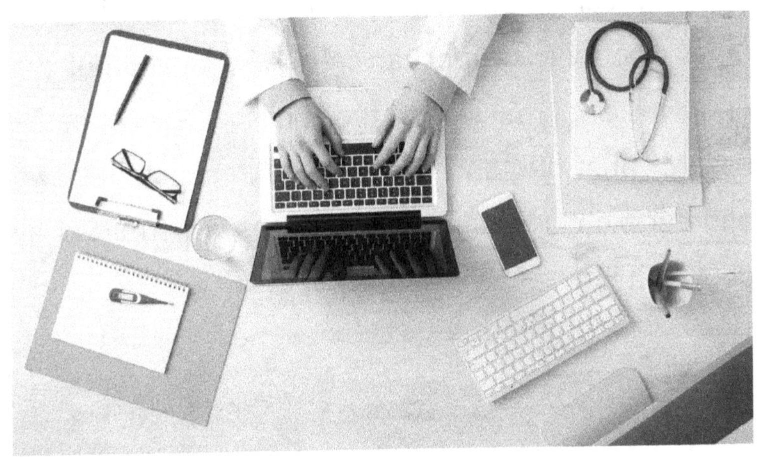

How to Increase or decrease Your Changes

TABLE OF CONTENTS

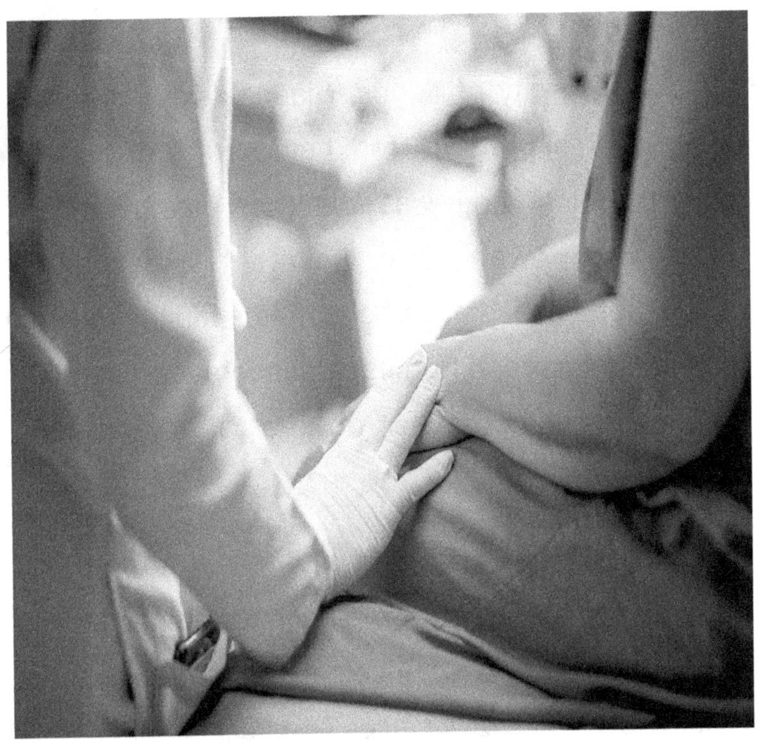

INTRODUCTION

In the vibrant city of Lagos, Nigeria, lived a woman named Sarah. Known for her warm smile and generous spirit, Sarah was a beloved member of her community. However, her lifestyle had become a source of concern. She often found herself consuming fast food from local vendors and spending long hours sitting at her desk or in front of the television.

One day, during a community health fair, Sarah attended a seminar on cancer awareness. The speaker, a renowned oncologist, emphasized the impact of lifestyle choices on cancer risk. He explained how regular physical activity and a balanced diet rich in fruits, vegetables, and whole grains could significantly reduce the risk of developing cancer. Conversely, a sedentary lifestyle and a diet high in processed foods and red meat could increase the risk.

Inspired by what she had learned, Sarah decided to make some changes. She started by visiting the local market more frequently, where she bought fresh produce such as okra, tomatoes, and leafy greens. She began preparing traditional dishes like efo riro and yam porridge, incorporating plenty of vegetables and reducing the amount of red meat.

Sarah also embraced physical activity. She joined a local dance group that met every morning for aerobic sessions infused with traditional Nigerian music. These sessions not only helped her stay active but also connected her with her cultural roots and community.

Over time, Sarah noticed significant improvements in her health. She felt more energetic, her weight was more manageable, and her mood improved. Her friends and family, inspired by her transformation, began adopting similar changes in their own lives.

Sarah's journey became a beacon of hope and inspiration in Lagos. She started organizing community events to raise awareness about the importance of a healthy lifestyle in cancer prevention. She invited health experts to speak, organized cooking classes focusing on nutritious meals, and led group exercise sessions.

Sarah's efforts paid off as the community of Lagos began to see the benefits of these lifestyle changes. People became more conscious of their eating habits and physical activity levels, fostering a healthier environment for everyone.

In the end, Sarah's story was a testament to the power of knowledge and the impact of lifestyle choices on health. Through her dedication and example, she helped create a wave of positive change, reducing cancer risk and enhancing the quality of life for many in her beloved city.

Cancer is a complex disease influenced by a multitude of factors, including genetics, environment, and lifestyle choices. Understanding the role of lifestyle factors is crucial in both preventing and managing cancer. Choices related to diet, physical activity, smoking, alcohol consumption, and exposure to certain environmental toxins can significantly impact cancer risk. By exploring how these factors can either increase or decrease the likelihood of developing cancer, individuals can make informed decisions to improve their overall health and reduce their cancer risk.

CHAPTER ONE: UNDERSTANDING CANCER AND ITS RISK FACTORS

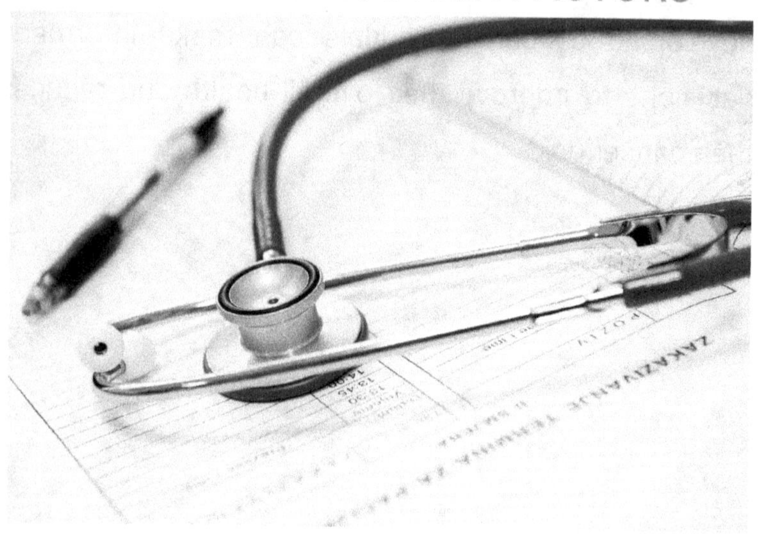

The complex disease that is characterized by the uncontrolled growth and spread of abnormal cells is called cancer. It can develop in virtually any part of the body and affects millions of people worldwide. While genetic predispositions play a significant role in cancer development, various lifestyle factors also contribute to either increasing or decreasing the risk. Understanding these factors is essential for prevention and early intervention. Key lifestyle elements such as diet, physical activity, smoking, alcohol consumption, and environmental exposures can all influence cancer risk. By making informed choices in these areas, individuals can take proactive steps towards reducing their likelihood of developing cancer and promoting overall health.

Cancer risk factors are varied and can include both non-modifiable and modifiable elements. Understanding these factors can help in prevention and early detection. Here are the primary risk factors for cancer:

Non-Modifiable Risk Factors

Non-modifiable risk factors for cancer are those elements that individuals cannot change or control. These factors are intrinsic to an individual and often arise from genetic, biological, or historical contexts.

Understanding these risk factors is crucial for identifying individuals at higher risk and developing targeted prevention and treatment strategies. Here are the main non-modifiable risk factors for cancer:

1. **Age**: Age is one of the most significant non-modifiable risk factors for cancer. The risk of developing cancer increases as individuals grow older. This is largely due to the accumulation of genetic mutations over time, a decline in the effectiveness of DNA repair mechanisms, and a weakened immune system. For instance, the median age for cancer diagnosis is around 66 years, meaning that half of the cases occur in people above this age.

2. **Gender**: Certain types of cancer have different prevalence rates between genders due to biological differences. For example, prostate cancer is exclusive to men, while breast cancer occurs significantly more often in women, although men can also develop it. Hormonal differences and reproductive factors often underlie these disparities.

3. Genetics and Family History: Genetic predisposition plays a crucial role in the risk of developing certain cancers. Some individuals inherit mutations in specific genes that significantly increase their cancer risk. For example, mutations in the BRCA1 and BRCA2 genes greatly elevate the risk of breast and ovarian cancers. A family history of cancer can indicate a potential inherited genetic risk, especially if close relatives were diagnosed with cancer at a young age.

4. Ethnicity and Race: Ethnicity and race can influence cancer risk due to genetic, environmental, and lifestyle factors unique to different populations. For instance, African American men have a higher risk of prostate cancer compared to men of other races. Similarly, certain genetic mutations that increase cancer risk may be more prevalent in specific ethnic groups, such as the BRCA1 and BRCA2 mutations in Ashkenazi Jewish populations.

5. Personal Medical History: A personal history of certain medical conditions can increase the risk of

cancer. For example, individuals who have had previous cancers are at higher risk for developing new cancers, either due to genetic susceptibility, the effects of treatment, or the original cancers impact on the body. Additionally, conditions like chronic inflammatory diseases, such as ulcerative colitis and Crohn's disease, can increase the risk of colorectal cancer.

6. Exposure to Certain Environmental Factors: While some environmental exposures can be controlled or avoided, certain early-life exposures or involuntary exposures constitute non-modifiable risks. For instance, exposure to radiation from medical treatments in childhood, atomic bomb survivors, or individuals exposed to high levels of radon gas may have an increased risk of certain types of cancer later in life.

7. Reproductive and Menstrual History

For women, certain reproductive and menstrual factors that are largely beyond their control can influence cancer risk. Early onset of menstruation (before age 12) and late menopause (after age 55) increase the risk of breast and endometrial cancers due to prolonged exposure to estrogen and progesterone. Understanding these non-modifiable risk factors underscores the importance of regular screenings and vigilant monitoring for individuals who may be at higher risk due to their age, genetics, or other intrinsic factors. While these risk factors cannot be changed, early detection and preventive strategies can significantly mitigate their impact on cancer development and progression.

Modifiable Risk Factors

Modifiable risk factors for cancer are lifestyle and environmental factors that individuals can change to reduce their risk of developing cancer. Here is a comprehensive overview:

1. Lifestyle Factors;

Tobacco Use

Smoking: Cigarette smoking is the leading cause of lung cancer and is linked to cancers of the mouth, throat, esophagus, pancreas, bladder, cervix, and kidney.

Secondhand Smoke: Exposure to secondhand smoke also increases cancer risk.

Cessation: Quitting smoking reduces the risk of developing and dying from cancer, even for long-term smokers.

Diet and Nutrition

Unhealthy Diet: Diets high in processed meats, red meats, and foods high in fat and low in fruits and vegetables can increase the risk of colorectal, stomach, and other cancers.

Healthy Eating: Consuming a diet rich in fruits, vegetables, whole grains, and lean proteins can help protect against cancer. Antioxidants and other nutrients in these foods have been shown to reduce cancer risk.

Physical Activity

Sedentary Lifestyle: Lack of physical activity is associated with an increased risk of colon, breast, and endometrial cancers.

Regular Exercise: Engaging in regular physical activity helps maintain a healthy weight and can reduce the risk of various cancers.

Alcohol Consumption

Excessive Drinking: Alcohol consumption is linked to an increased risk of cancers of the mouth, throat, esophagus, liver, colon, and breast.

Moderation: Limiting alcohol intake can reduce these risks. The recommended limits are up to one drink per day for women and up to two drinks per day for men.

2. Environmental Factors;

Exposure to Carcinogens

Occupational Hazards: Exposure to carcinogens such as asbestos, benzene, and certain dyes in the workplace can increase cancer risk.

Pollution: Air pollution and exposure to chemicals like radon and formaldehyde can increase lung and other cancer risks.

3. Behavioral Factors;

Sun Exposure

Ultraviolet (UV) Radiation: Excessive exposure to UV radiation from the sun and tanning beds increases the risk of skin cancers, including melanoma.

Protection: Using sunscreen, wearing protective clothing, and avoiding peak sun hours can help reduce this risk.

Infections.

Human Papillomavirus (HPV): HPV infection is a major risk factor for cervical, anal, and some head and neck cancers.

Hepatitis B and C: These infections increase the risk of liver cancer.

Prevention: Vaccination against HPV and hepatitis B, practicing safe sex, and avoiding sharing needles can reduce these infection-related cancer risks.

4. Preventive Health Measures

Regular Screenings

Lack of Screening: Not participating in regular cancer screenings can delay diagnosis and treatment.

Early Detection: Regular screenings for cancers such as breast, cervical, colorectal, and prostate can detect cancer early, when it is most treatable.

Vaccinations

HPV Vaccine: Vaccination against HPV can prevent cervical and other HPV-related cancers.

Hepatitis B Vaccine: This vaccine can reduce the risk of developing liver cancer.

5. Socioeconomic Factors

Education and Awareness

Lack of Knowledge: Poor understanding of cancer risks and prevention methods can lead to unhealthy behaviors.

Health Education: Increased awareness and education about cancer prevention can empower individuals to make healthier choices and seek regular medical care.

Access to Healthcare

Limited Access: Poor access to healthcare services can delay cancer detection and treatment.

Improved Access: Enhancing access to healthcare ensures timely screenings, vaccinations, and treatments, improving cancer outcomes.

By addressing these modifiable risk factors, individuals can significantly reduce their risk of developing cancer. Public health initiatives, personal lifestyle changes, and regular medical care all play crucial roles in cancer prevention.

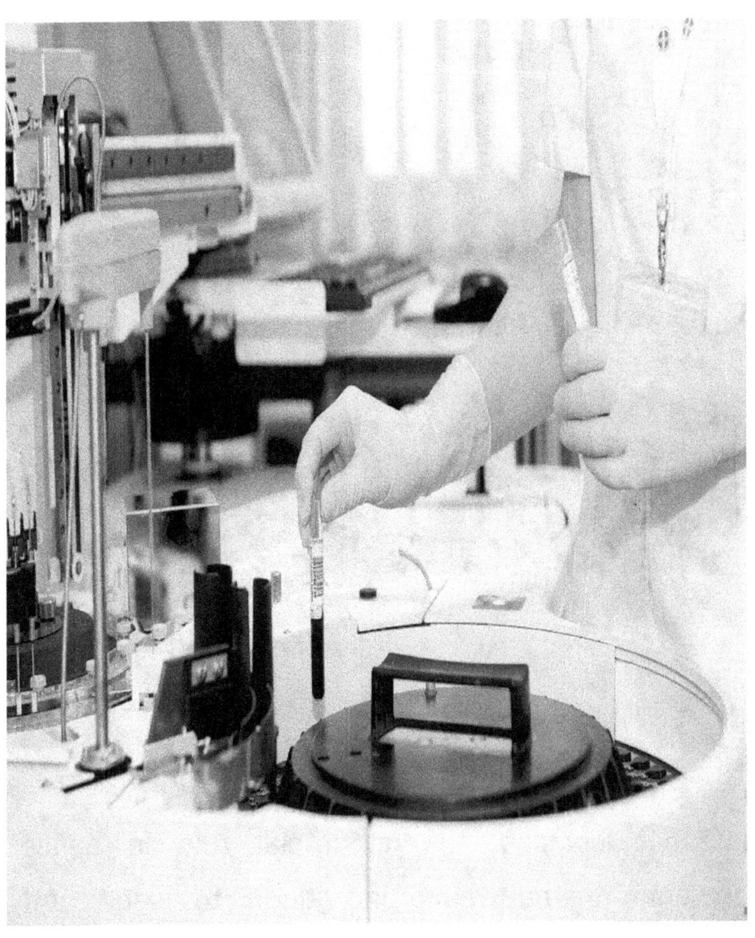

CHAPTER TWO: THE IMPORTANCE OF LIFESTYLE IN CANCER PREVENTION

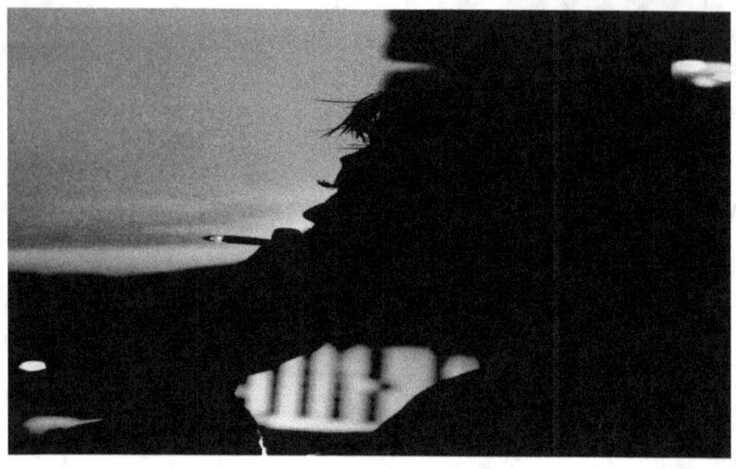

Lifestyle choices play a crucial role in cancer prevention, empowering individuals to significantly reduce their risk through informed decisions and healthy habits. While genetics and environmental exposures are important factors, many aspects of lifestyle are within personal control and can have a profound impact on cancer risk.

Understanding how these elements contribute to cancer prevention can empower individuals to make healthier choices that reduce their risk of developing the disease.

Diet and Nutrition

A healthy diet plays a critical role in cancer prevention. Diets rich in fruits, vegetables, whole grains, and lean proteins provide essential nutrients and antioxidants that can protect cells from damage. Key dietary recommendations include:

1. High Fiber Intake: Consuming plenty of fruits, vegetables, and whole grains helps maintain a healthy digestive system and may reduce the risk of colorectal cancer.

2. Low Red and Processed Meat Consumption: Limiting red and processed meats can lower the risk of colorectal and stomach cancers. These meats can contain carcinogenic compounds that form during processing or cooking.

3. Healthy Fats: Choosing sources of healthy fats, such as those from fish, nuts, and olive oil, over saturated and trans fats, which are linked to increased cancer risk.

4. Moderate Sugar and Salt: Reducing intake of sugar and salt can help prevent obesity and hypertension, both of which are associated with increased cancer risk.

Physical Activity

Regular physical activity is associated with a lower risk of several types of cancer, including breast, colorectal, and endometrial cancers. Exercise helps maintain a healthy weight, regulates hormones, and enhances the immune system. Recommendations include:

1. Moderate to Vigorous Activity: Engaging in at least 150 minutes of moderate-intensity or 75 minutes of vigorous-intensity exercise per week.

2. Strength Training: Incorporating muscle-

strengthening activities at least twice a week.

Tobacco Use

Tobacco use is the leading preventable cause of cancer. It is linked to various cancers, including lung, mouth, throat, esophagus, and bladder cancers. Quitting smoking and avoiding secondhand smoke are critical measures for cancer prevention. Key points include:

1. Smoking Cessation: Programs and medications can help individuals quit smoking, significantly reducing cancer risk.

2. Avoiding Smokeless Tobacco: Products like chewing tobacco are also carcinogenic.

Alcohol Consumption

Alcohol consumption is linked to an increased risk of several cancers, including those of the mouth, throat, esophagus, liver, breast, and colon. The risk increases with the amount of alcohol consumed. Recommendations for cancer prevention include:

1. Limiting Alcohol Intake: If alcohol is consumed, it should be done in moderation—up to one drink per day for women and two drinks per day for men.

Un Exposure and UV Radiation

Excessive sun exposure and the use of tanning beds are major risk factors for skin cancer, including melanoma. Protective measures include:

1. Using Sunscreen: Applying broad-spectrum sunscreen with an SPF of 30 or higher.

2. Protective Clothing: Wearing hats, sunglasses, and long-sleeved clothing when exposed to the sun.

3. Avoiding Tanning Beds: Steering clear of artificial sources of UV radiation.

Weight Management

Maintaining a healthy weight is crucial for cancer prevention. Obesity is linked to an increased risk of several cancers, including breast, prostate, pancreatic, and colorectal cancers. Strategies for maintaining a healthy weight include:

1. **Balanced Diet**: Eating nutrient-dense foods and managing portion sizes.

2. **Regular Exercise**: Combining aerobic activity with strength training.

Preventive Healthcare

Regular screening and preventive healthcare can detect cancers early when they are most treatable. Vaccinations, such as the HPV vaccine, can prevent infections that cause cancer. Regular check-ups and following recommended screening guidelines for cancers like breast, cervical, and colorectal can significantly improve outcomes.

Stress Management and Mental Health

Chronic stress and poor mental health can indirectly contribute to cancer risk by leading to unhealthy behaviors such as smoking, excessive drinking, and overeating. Strategies include:

1. Stress Reduction Techniques: Practices like mindfulness, meditation, and yoga.

2. Social Support: Building a strong network of family and friends.

3. Professional Help: Seeking therapy or counseling when needed.

A healthy lifestyle is a powerful tool in cancer prevention.

CHAPTER THREE: UNDERSTANDING YOUR DIAGNOSIS

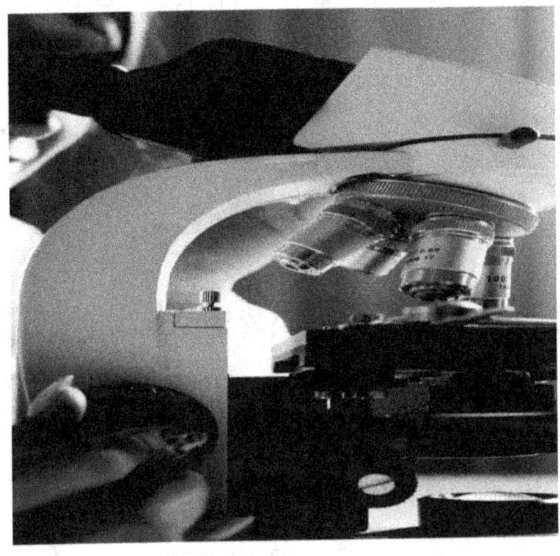

Understanding your diagnosis is a critical first step for cancer patients in navigating their treatment and managing their health. A cancer diagnosis can be overwhelming, but gaining a clear understanding of what it means can help patients make informed decisions about their care.

1. Initial Symptoms and Tests: Diagnosis often begins when a patient presents with symptoms that could be indicative of cancer. These symptoms can vary widely depending on the type of cancer. Initial tests may include blood tests, imaging (such as X-rays, CT scans, MRI), and physical exams.

2. Biopsy and Pathology: If imaging or other tests suggest cancer, a biopsy is typically performed. A biopsy involves taking a small sample of tissue from the suspected cancer site. This sample is then examined under a microscope by a pathologist, who determines whether cancer cells are present and identifies the type of cancer.

3. Staging: Once cancer is confirmed, staging is conducted to determine the extent of the disease. This involves additional imaging tests and possibly further biopsies to see if cancer has spread (metastasized) to other parts of the body. Staging is critical for planning treatment and predicting outcomes. It ranges from Stage 0 (in situ, or localized)

to Stage IV (metastasized).

Communicating with Healthcare Providers.

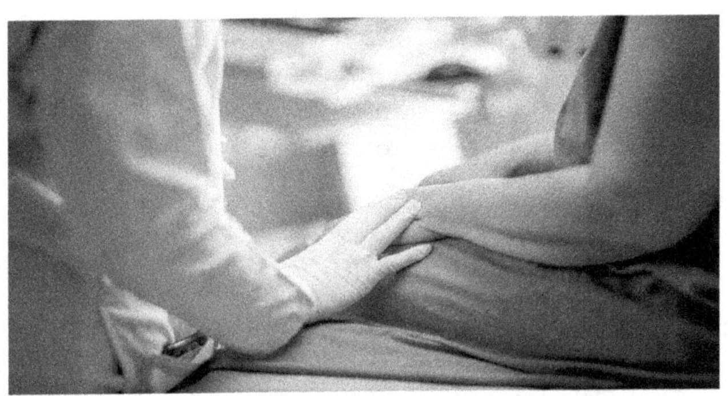

1. Questions to Ask: Patients should feel empowered to ask their healthcare providers about their diagnosis. Important questions might include:

What type of cancer do I have?

What stage is my cancer, and what does that mean?

What are my treatment options, and what are the benefits and risks of each?

What is my prognosis?

2. Second Opinions: It can be beneficial to seek a second opinion to confirm the diagnosis and explore all treatment options. This can be especially important in cases of rare or aggressive cancers.

3. Support Systems: Having a support system in place is vital. This includes family, friends, support groups, and mental health professionals who can help manage the emotional and psychological impacts of a cancer diagnosis.

Treatment Planning

1. Multidisciplinary Approach: Treatment often involves a team of specialists, including oncologists, surgeons, radiologists, and nurses. Each plays a role in developing and implementing a comprehensive treatment plan.

2. Treatment Options: Depending on the type and stage of cancer, treatment options may include surgery, chemotherapy, radiation therapy, immunotherapy, targeted therapy, or a combination of these.

3. Clinical Trials: For some patients, participating in clinical trials can provide access to new and experimental treatments that are not yet widely available.

Managing Information and Decisions

1. Educational Resources: Utilizing reliable sources of information can help patients understand their diagnosis and treatment options. Resources like the American Cancer Society, National Cancer Institute, and other reputable cancer organizations provide comprehensive and up-to-date information.

2. Decision-Making: It is crucial for patients to take an active role in their treatment decisions. This involves understanding the risks and benefits of each option and considering personal values and preferences.

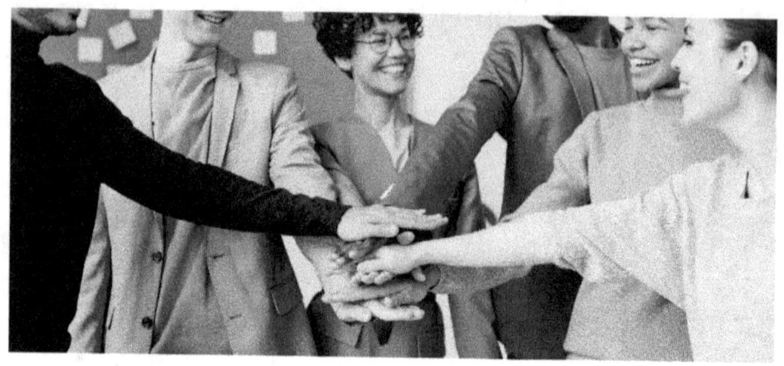

1.Counseling and Therapy: Professional counseling can help patients cope with the stress, anxiety, and depression that may accompany a cancer diagnosis.

2. Support Groups: Joining a support group can provide a sense of community and understanding, offering a space to share experiences and advice.

Understanding your cancer diagnosis is a multifaceted process that involves grasping the medical aspects of the disease, communicating effectively with healthcare providers, exploring treatment options, and finding emotional and psychological support. By becoming well-informed and actively involved in their care, patients can better navigate the challenges of a cancer diagnosis and treatment.

Different types of cancer

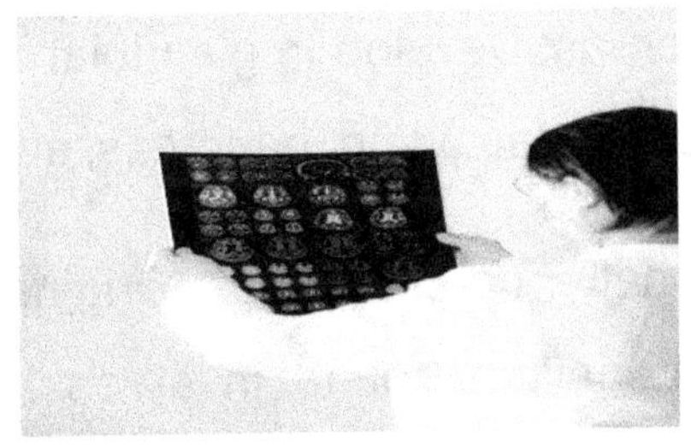

Cancer is a broad term for a collection of diseases characterized by uncontrolled cell growth, invasion into surrounding tissues, and sometimes metastasis, where cancer cells spread to other parts of the body. There are over 100 types of cancer, typically categorized by the type of cell or tissue from which they originate. Here are some of the main types of cancer:

1. Carcinomas

Carcinomas are the most common type of cancer. They arise from the epithelial cells that line the inside and outside surfaces of the body. Carcinomas can be further divided into several subtypes:

Adenocarcinomas: Develop in glandular tissues, such as the breast, prostate, lung, pancreas, and colon.

Squamous cell carcinomas: Originate in the squamous epithelium, found in areas like the skin, lungs, and lining of the digestive tract.

Basal cell carcinomas:

A type of skin cancer that arises from the basal cells in the epidermis.

2. Sarcomas

Sarcomas originate in the connective and supportive tissues, such as bones, muscles, fat, and cartilage. Common types include:

Osteosarcoma: Starts in bone cells.

Chondrosarcoma: Arises in cartilage cells.

Liposarcoma: Develops in fat cells.

Leiomyosarcoma: Originates in smooth muscle cells.

3. Leukemias

Leukemias are cancers of the blood or bone marrow, characterized by an overproduction of abnormal white blood cells. They are classified based on the speed of progression (acute or chronic) and the type of blood cell affected (lymphocytic or myeloid):

Acute lymphocytic leukemia (ALL): Rapidly progressing cancer that affects lymphoid cells.

Chronic lymphocytic leukemia (CLL): Slower-progressing cancer affecting lymphoid cells.

Acute myeloid leukemia (AML): Rapidly progressing cancer that affects myeloid cells.

Chronic myeloid leukemia (CML): Slower-progressing cancer affecting myeloid cells.

4. Lymphomas

Lymphomas are cancers of the lymphatic system, which is part of the immune system. There are two main types:

Hodgkin lymphoma (Hodgkin's disease): Characterized by the presence of Reed-Sternberg cells.

Non-Hodgkin lymphoma: A diverse group of lymphatic cancers not featuring Reed-Sternberg cells, further classified into B-cell and T-cell lymphomas.

5. Myeloma

Multiple myeloma is a cancer that originates in the plasma cells of the bone marrow, which are a type of white blood cell responsible for producing antibodies.

6. Melanoma

Melanoma is a type of skin cancer that originates in melanocytes, the cells that produce the pigment melanin. It is less common than basal and squamous cell skin cancers but is more dangerous due to its tendency to spread.

7. Central Nervous System Cancers

These cancers originate in the brain and spinal cord. They include:

Gliomas: Tumors that arise from glial cells.

Meningiomas: Tumors that develop from the meninges, the protective membranes covering the brain and spinal cord.

8. Germ Cell Tumors

These tumors arise from the cells that give rise to sperm or eggs. They typically occur in the testes or ovaries but can also appear in other parts of the body.

9. Neuroendocrine Tumors

These cancers develop from cells that release hormones into the blood in response to a signal from the nervous system. They can occur in various organs, including the lungs and gastrointestinal tract. A well-known subtype is carcinoid tumors.

10. Rare Cancers

There are numerous other rare types of cancer, each affecting different tissues and organs. Examples include:

Merkel cell carcinoma: A rare and aggressive skin cancer.

Kaposi's sarcoma: Often associated with HIV infection, this cancer forms in the lining of blood and lymph vessels.

Cancer Staging and Grading

Understanding cancer staging and grading is essential for determining the extent of the disease, planning treatment, and predicting outcomes. Here is a detailed explanation of both concepts:

Cancer Staging

Cancer staging describes the size of the primary tumor and whether it has spread to other parts of the body. It is crucial for planning treatment and predicting prognosis.

TNM System

The most commonly used staging system is the TNM system, which stands for Tumor, Nodes, and Metastasis:

1. Tumor (T):

TX: Primary tumor cannot be evaluated.

T0: No evidence of primary tumor.

Tis: Carcinoma in situ (early cancer that has not spread to neighboring tissue).

T1-T4: Size and/or extent of the primary tumor. Higher numbers indicate a larger tumor or greater extent.

2. Nodes (N):

NX: Regional lymph nodes cannot be evaluated.

N0: No regional lymph node involvement.

N1-N3: Involvement of regional lymph nodes. Higher

numbers indicate more extensive involvement.

3. Metastasis (M):

MX: Distant metastasis cannot be evaluated.

M0: No distant metastasis.

M1: Distant metastasis is present.

Stage Grouping

The TNM results are combined to determine an overall stage, ranging from 0 to IV:

Stage 0: Carcinoma in situ.

Stage I: Localized cancer, limited to the organ of origin.

Stage II: More advanced local disease, may involve nearby lymph nodes.

Stage III: Regional spread to surrounding tissues and possibly lymph nodes.

Stage IV: Distant metastasis, cancer has spread to

other parts of the body.

Cancer Grading

Cancer grading refers to how much cancer cells resemble normal cells under a microscope. It indicates how quickly the cancer is likely to grow and spread.

Grading Scale

1. Grade 1 (Low Grade):

Cells look more like normal cells (well-differentiated).

Tend to grow and spread slowly.

Better prognosis.

2. Grade 2 (Intermediate Grade):

Cells are moderately differentiated.

Have features between low and high grade.

3. Grade 3 (High Grade):

Cells look less like normal cells (poorly differentiated).

Tend to grow and spread more quickly.

Worse prognosis.

4.Grade 4 (Undifferentiated/Anaplastic):

Cells do not resemble normal cells at all (undifferentiated).

Highly aggressive and likely to spread quickly.

Specific Grading Systems

Different types of cancer have specific grading systems. For example:

Gleason Score for Prostate Cancer: Combines two grades of the most common patterns of cells, each graded from 1 to 5, resulting in a score ranging from 2 to 10.

Bloom-Richardson Grade for Breast Cancer:Evaluates tubule formation, nuclear grade, and mitotic rate to assign a grade.

Importance of Staging and Grading

1. Treatment Planning: Staging and grading help determine the most appropriate treatment options. Early-stage and low-grade cancers might be treated with surgery alone, while more advanced or higher-grade cancers might require additional treatments like chemotherapy, radiation, or targeted therapies.

2. Prognosis: Provides information about the likely course and outcome of the disease. Early-stage and low-grade cancers generally have a better prognosis compared to late-stage and high-grade cancers.

3. Clinical Trials: Helps identify suitable candidates for clinical trials that test new treatments.

Communicating with Healthcare Providers

Patients should discuss the implications of their cancer's stage and grade with their healthcare providers to understand their specific situation better. Questions to ask might include:

What is the stage and grade of my cancer?

How do these factors influence my treatment options

and prognosis?

Are there clinical trials available for my stage and grade of cancer?

Cancer staging and grading are fundamental aspects of understanding the nature of the disease, guiding treatment decisions, and predicting outcomes. By comprehending these concepts, patients and healthcare providers can work together to develop an effective and personalized treatment plan.

Common Symptoms and Warning Signs

Cancer can manifest in a wide variety of symptoms, often depending on the type and location of the cancer. However, there are several common symptoms and warning signs that can indicate the presence of cancer. It's important to note that these symptoms can also be caused by conditions other than cancer, but persistent or unusual symptoms should be evaluated by a healthcare professional.

1. **Unexplained Weight Loss:** Many people with cancer will experience significant weight loss without trying. Losing 10 pounds or more may be one of the first signs of cancer, particularly cancers of the pancreas, stomach, esophagus, or lung.

2. **Fever:** Fever is common, especially if the cancer or its treatment affects the immune system. It often happens in cases of leukemia or lymphoma.

3. **Fatigue:** Extreme tiredness that doesn't improve with rest can be an important symptom. It may be related to cancers like leukemia, colon, or stomach cancer.

4. **Pain:** Pain can be an early symptom with some cancers like bone cancer or testicular cancer. A headache that does not go away or respond to treatment can be a symptom of a brain tumor.

5. **Skin Changes:** In addition to cancers of the skin, some internal cancers can produce visible skin changes such as darker looking skin

(hyperpigmentation), yellowish skin and eyes (jaundice), reddened skin (erythema), itching, or excessive hair growth.

Specific Symptoms

1. Changes in Bowel or Bladder Habits: Long-term constipation, diarrhea, or a change in the size of the stool may be a sign of colon cancer. Pain when passing urine, blood in the urine, or a change in bladder function (such as needing to pass urine more or less often) could be related to bladder or prostate cancer.

2. Sores that Do Not Heal: A persistent sore in the mouth could be an oral cancer, especially in people who smoke or frequently drink alcohol. Sores on the penis or vagina may be signs of infection or an early cancer.

3. White Patches Inside the Mouth or White Spots on the Tongue: These can be leukoplakia, a precancerous area that is caused by frequent irritation and can be caused by smoking or other tobacco use.

4. Unusual Bleeding or Discharge: Unusual bleeding can occur in early or advanced cancer. Coughing up blood can be a sign of lung cancer. Blood in the stool (which can look like very dark or black stool) could be a sign of colon or rectal cancer. Women with cancer of the cervix or the endometrium (lining of the uterus) may have abnormal vaginal bleeding. Blood in the urine can be a sign of bladder or kidney cancer.

5. Thickening or Lump in the Breast or Other Parts of the Body: Many cancers can be felt through the skin. These cancers occur mostly in the breast, testicle, lymph nodes (glands), and the soft tissues of the body. A lump or thickening may be an early or late sign of cancer.

6. Indigestion or Trouble Swallowing: Persistent indigestion or difficulty swallowing can be a sign of cancer of the esophagus, stomach, or throat.

7. Recent Change in a Wart or Mole or Any New Skin Change: Any wart, mole, or freckle that changes color, size, or shape, or that loses its sharp border, may be

melanoma or another skin cancer.

8. Nagging Cough or Hoarseness: A cough that does not go away may be a sign of lung cancer. Hoarseness can be a sign of cancer of the larynx (voice box) or thyroid gland.

When to See a Doctor

While these symptoms can be caused by other conditions, it is important to see a healthcare provider if they persist for more than a couple of weeks or if they are particularly severe. Early detection and diagnosis can significantly improve treatment outcomes for many cancers. Regular screenings and being aware of your body changes are crucial for early detection.

Treatment

Cancer treatment varies widely based on the type, stage, and location of the cancer, as well as the patient's overall health. Common treatments include:

1. Surgery: Removal of the tumor and surrounding

tissues.

2. **Radiation therapy:** Using high-energy radiation to kill cancer cells.

3. **Chemotherapy:** Drugs that kill or slow the growth of cancer cells.

4. **Targeted therapy:** Drugs or other substances that specifically target cancer cells with less damage to normal cells.

5. **Immunotherapy:** Boosts the body's natural defenses to fight cancer.

6. **Hormone therapy:** Used for cancers that are sensitive to hormones, like some breast and prostate cancers.

Understanding the specifics of each cancer type helps in tailoring the most effective treatment approaches and improving patient outcomes.

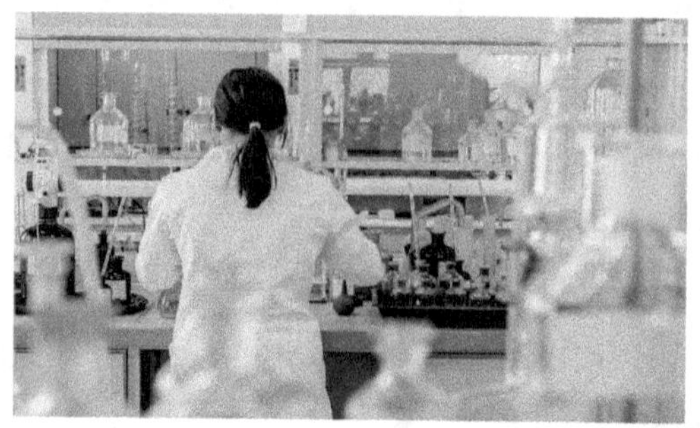

CHAPTER FOUR:

FACTORS THAT INCREASE CANCER RISK.

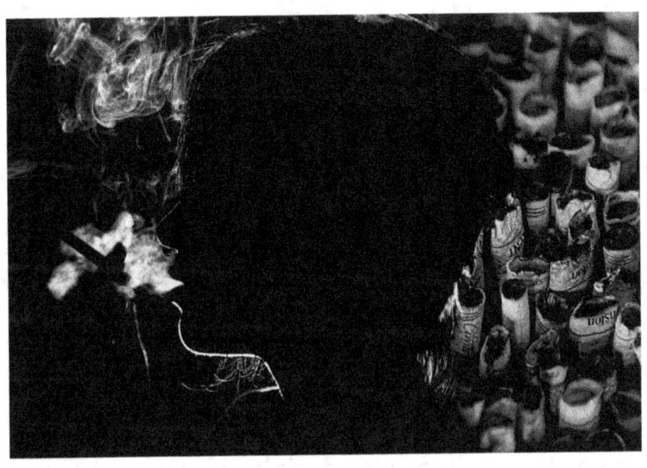

Cancer risk is influenced by a variety of factors, which can broadly be categorized into lifestyle choices, environmental exposures, and genetic predispositions. Here are some key factors that increase the risk of developing cancer:

Lifestyle Choices

1. Tobacco Use: Smoking and using other forms of tobacco are the leading causes of various cancers, particularly lung cancer, as well as cancers of the mouth, throat, pancreas, and bladder.

2. Diet and Nutrition: A diet high in red and processed meats, low in fruits and vegetables, or high in processed and sugary foods can increase the risk of cancers such as colorectal cancer.

3. Physical Inactivity: Lack of regular physical activity is linked to an increased risk of several cancers, including breast and colon cancer.

4. Alcohol Consumption: Excessive alcohol intake is associated with a higher risk of cancers of the liver, breast, mouth, throat, and esophagus.

5. Obesity: Being overweight or obese is linked to an increased risk of various cancers, including breast, colorectal, endometrial, and pancreatic cancer.

1. Radiation: Exposure to high levels of radiation, including ultraviolet (UV) radiation from the sun and radon gas, can increase the risk of skin cancer and lung cancer, respectively.

2. Carcinogenic Chemicals: Contact with certain chemicals, such as asbestos, benzene, and formaldehyde, can elevate the risk of cancers like mesothelioma, leukemia, and other types of cancer.

3. Air Pollution: Long-term exposure to polluted air, especially in urban areas with high traffic or industrial emissions, is linked to increased lung cancer risk.

4. Infections: Some viruses and bacteria, such as human papillomavirus (HPV), hepatitis B and C, and Helicobacter pylori, are associated with a higher risk of cancers such as cervical, liver, and stomach cancer.

Genetic Factors

1. Family History: A family history of certain cancers can increase an individual's risk due to shared genetic

mutations and environmental factors.

2. Inherited Genetic Mutations: Certain inherited mutations, such as BRCA1 and BRCA2, significantly increase the risk of breast and ovarian cancers.

3. Genetic Syndromes: Conditions like Lynch syndrome and Li-Fraumeni syndrome are linked to a higher risk of various cancers due to specific genetic abnormalities.

Understanding these risk factors can help individuals make informed lifestyle choices and seek appropriate medical screening and interventions to reduce their cancer risk. By addressing modifiable factors and being aware of genetic predispositions, the overall incidence of cancer can be mitigated.

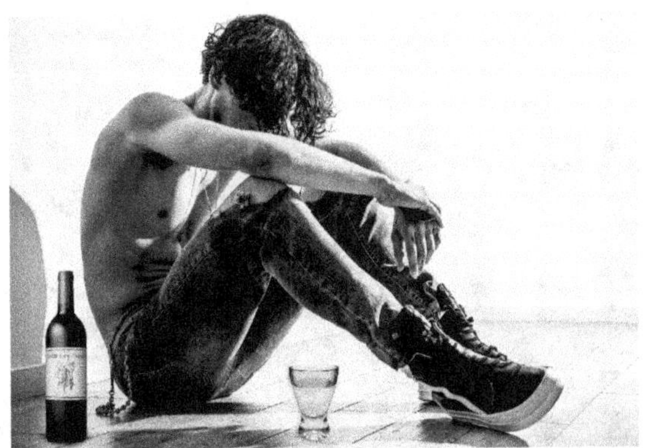

CHAPTER FIVE: FACTORS THAT DECREASE CANCER RISK.

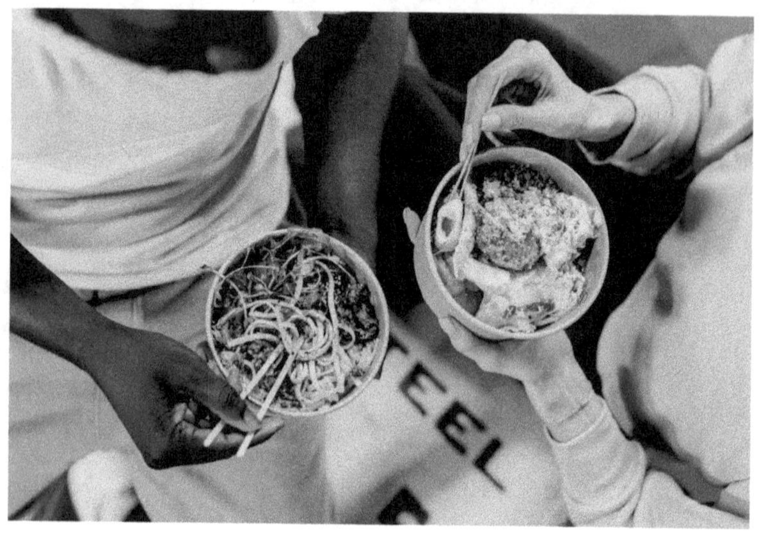

Reducing cancer risk involves a combination of lifestyle choices, environmental factors, and preventive healthcare. Here are several key factors that can decrease the risk of developing cancer:

Healthy Diet:

1. Fruits and Vegetables: High intake of a variety of fruits and vegetables provides essential vitamins, minerals, and antioxidants that help protect cells from damage.

2. Whole Grains and Fiber: Consuming whole grains and dietary fiber can reduce the risk of colorectal cancer.

3. Limit Processed and Red Meat: Reducing intake of processed meats and red meats is associated with a lower risk of colorectal cancer.

Regular Physical Activity:

Engaging in regular physical activity helps maintain a healthy weight and reduces the risk of several types of cancer, including breast, prostate, lung, and colon cancer.

Maintaining a Healthy Weight:

Obesity is linked to an increased risk of various cancers, including breast, prostate, lung, colon, and kidney cancer. Maintaining a healthy weight through diet and exercise can reduce this risk.

Avoiding Tobacco:

Tobacco use is the leading cause of lung cancer and is also associated with cancers of the mouth, throat, pancreas, bladder, cervix, and kidney. Avoiding tobacco in all forms reduces cancer risk significantly.

Limiting Alcohol Consumption:

Excessive alcohol consumption is linked to an increased risk of cancers of the mouth, throat, esophagus, liver, breast, and colon. Limiting alcohol intake can reduce this risk.

Protecting Skin from Sun Exposure:

Using sunscreen, wearing protective clothing, and avoiding excessive sun exposure reduces the risk of skin cancers, including melanoma.

Vaccination:

Vaccines like the Human Papillomavirus (HPV) vaccine can prevent cervical and other HPV-related cancers. The Hepatitis B vaccine can lower the risk of liver cancer.

Avoiding Risky Behaviors:

Practicing safe sex and avoiding sharing needles can prevent infections with viruses such as HPV and HIV, which are linked to certain cancers.

Regular Medical Screenings:

Regular screenings can detect cancers early when they are most treatable. Screenings for breast, cervical, colorectal, and skin cancers are particularly important.

Minimizing Exposure to Environmental Toxins:

Limiting exposure to known carcinogens in the environment, such as asbestos, radon, and certain chemicals, can reduce cancer risk.

Healthy Sleep Patterns:

Maintaining a regular sleep schedule and ensuring adequate sleep may help reduce cancer risk, as disrupted circadian rhythms have been linked to certain types of cancer.

Stress Management:

Stress Management:

Chronic stress can impact the immune system and other bodily functions. Managing stress through techniques like mindfulness, exercise, and relaxation can contribute to overall health and potentially reduce cancer risk.

By incorporating these strategies, individuals can significantly lower their risk of developing cancer and improve their overall health and well-being.

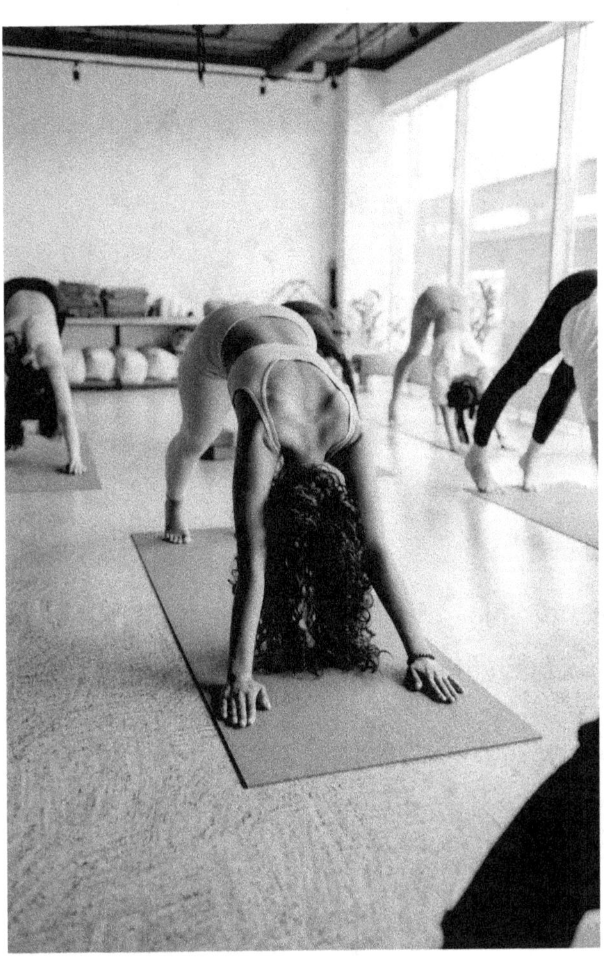

CHAPTER SIX: PRACTICAL TIPS FOR A HEALTHIER LIFESTYLE

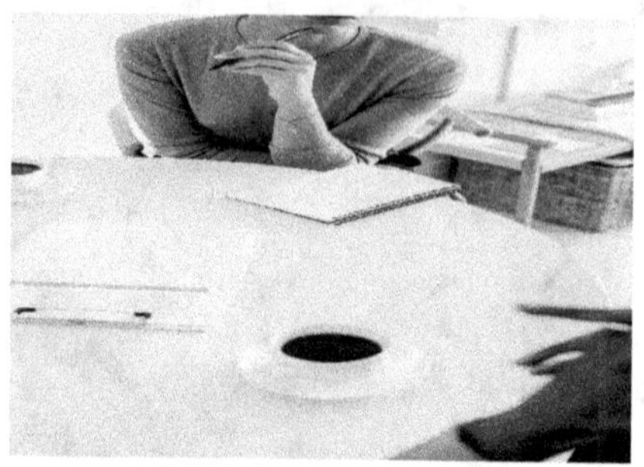

Adopting a healthier lifestyle can play a significant role in cancer prevention and overall well-being.

By integrating these practical tips into your daily routine, you can significantly reduce your risk of cancer and improve your overall health and quality of life. Here are some comprehensive, practical tips:

Creating a Balanced Diet Plan

Creating a balanced diet plan for cancer patients requires careful consideration of their specific needs, treatment plans, and side effects they may be experiencing. Here Is a guide to developing such a diet plan:

Key Principles:

1. **Personalization**: Tailor the diet to the individual's specific cancer type, treatment stage, nutritional status, and personal preferences.

2. **Nutrient Density**: Focus on foods high in vitamins, minerals, protein, and calories to support overall health and recovery.

3. **Hydration**: Ensure adequate fluid intake to prevent dehydration, especially important during treatments like chemotherapy and radiation.

Components of a Balanced Diet:

1. Proteins

Importance: Helps repair tissues, maintain muscle mass, and support the immune system.

Sources: Lean meats, poultry, fish, eggs, dairy

products, beans, legumes, nuts, and seeds.

2. Carbohydrates

Importance: Provide energy, especially important if the patient experiences fatigue.

Sources: Whole grains (brown rice, quinoa, whole wheat bread), fruits, vegetables, and legumes.

3. Fats

Importance: Essential for energy, cell function, and absorbing fat-soluble vitamins.

Sources: Healthy fats like avocados, nuts, seeds, olive oil, and fatty fish (salmon, mackerel).

4. Vitamins and Minerals

Importance: Support immune function and overall health.

Sources: A variety of fruits and vegetables, whole grains, and fortified foods.

5. Fiber

Importance: Aids in digestion and prevents constipation.

Sources: Whole grains, fruits, vegetables, legumes, and nuts.

Sample Diet Plan:

Breakfast

Option 1: Oatmeal topped with berries, nuts, and a dollop of Greek yogurt.

Option 2: Smoothie with spinach, banana, protein powder, almond milk, and chia seeds.

Mid-Morning Snack

Option 1: Apple slices with peanut butter.

Option 2: Carrot sticks and hummus.

Lunch

Option 1: Grilled chicken salad with mixed greens, quinoa, avocado, and a vinaigrette dressing.

Option 2: Lentil soup with whole-grain bread.

Afternoon Snack

Option 1: Cottage cheese with pineapple chunks.

Option 2: Handful of mixed nuts and dried fruit.

Dinner

Option 1: Baked salmon with steamed broccoli and sweet potato.

Option 2: Stir-fried tofu with mixed vegetables and brown rice.

Evening Snack

Option 1: Greek yogurt with honey and almonds.

Option 2: Whole-grain crackers with cheese.

Special Considerations:

Side Effects Management: Adapt the diet to manage side effects of treatment (e.g., soft, bland foods for mouth sores, high-fiber foods for constipation, small, frequent meals for nausea).

Supplements: Consult with a healthcare provider about the need for supplements to address any deficiencies.

Food Safety: Prioritize food safety to avoid infections, particularly in patients with weakened immune systems (e.g., thoroughly cooking meats, avoiding raw or undercooked foods).

Hydration:

Encourage drinking water, herbal teas, and broths. Electrolyte solutions can be beneficial if dehydration is a concern due to vomiting or diarrhea.

Professional Guidance:

Regular consultations with a registered dietitian specialized in oncology nutrition can help in adjusting the diet plan as needed based on the patient's ongoing health status and treatment response.

This approach ensures that cancer patients receive

the necessary nutrients to support their treatment and recovery while addressing any specific challenges they may face.

Incorporating Exercise into Daily Routine

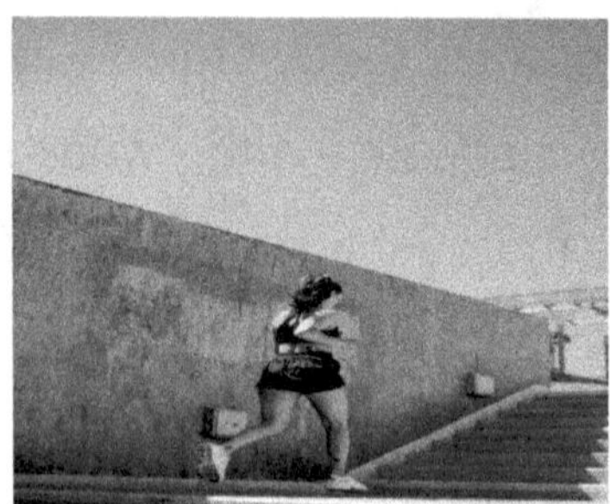

Incorporating exercise into your daily routine is a powerful way to promote a healthier lifestyle, particularly for those impacted by cancer. Here are some comprehensive tips to help you integrate physical activity into your everyday life:

1. Consult with Your Healthcare Provider

Personalized Plan: Ensure that any exercise regimen is safe and tailored to your specific health needs and current treatment plan.

Monitor Health: Regular check-ups to adjust your exercise plan based on your progress and any new health developments.

2. Start Slow and Build Gradually

Begin with Gentle Activities: Start with low-intensity exercises like walking, stretching, or gentle yoga.

Increase Intensity Gradually: As you build strength and endurance, slowly increase the intensity and duration of your workouts.

3. Incorporate Aerobic Exercise

Cardio Workouts: Engage in activities such as brisk walking, swimming, or cycling for at least 150 minutes per week.

Break It Up: Split exercise into shorter sessions (e.g., 30 minutes, 5 times a week) to make it more manageable.

4. Strength Training

Resistance Exercises: Use light weights, resistance bands, or body-weight exercises like squats and push-ups to build muscle strength.

Twice Weekly: Aim for at least two sessions per week, focusing on major muscle groups.

5. Flexibility and Balance

Stretching: Incorporate daily stretching exercises to improve flexibility and reduce stiffness.

Balance Exercises: Practice balance exercises, such as standing on one foot or tai chi, to enhance stability and prevent falls.

6. Incorporate Movement into Daily Activities

Active Commuting: Walk or cycle instead of driving when possible.

Household Chores: Use activities like gardening, cleaning, and climbing stairs as opportunities to move more.

Desk Exercises: If you have a sedentary job, take

breaks to stand, stretch, or walk around.

7. Join a Group or Class

Social Support: Join a fitness class or exercise group to stay motivated and accountable.

Specialized Classes: Look for programs designed for cancer survivors which can provide tailored support and encouragement.

8. Mind-Body Practices

Yoga and Pilates: These practices can improve both physical and mental well-being, combining gentle strength and flexibility exercises with relaxation techniques.

Meditation and Breathing Exercises: Integrate these into your routine to help manage stress and improve mental health.

9. Set Realistic Goals

Short-Term Milestones: Set achievable, short-term goals to build confidence and momentum.

Long-Term Objectives: Have broader health and fitness objectives to keep you focused and motivated over time.

10. Listen to Your Body

Rest When Needed: Pay attention to how your body feels and rest if you experience pain, fatigue, or other symptoms.

Adapt Workouts: Adjust your exercise routine based on your daily energy levels and physical condition.

11. Stay Hydrated and Eat Well

Hydration: Drink plenty of water before, during, and after exercise.

Nutrition: Maintain a balanced diet to support your exercise regimen and overall health.

12. Track Your Progress

Exercise Log: Keep a journal of your activities, noting what you did, how you felt, and any changes in your health.

By integrating these tips into your daily routine, you can enhance your physical health, improve your mood, and potentially aid in your recovery and overall well-being during and after cancer treatment.

Strategies for Reducing Stress

Managing stress is particularly crucial for individuals with cancer due to the physical and emotional toll of the disease and its treatments. Here are comprehensive strategies to help reduce stress:

Emotional and Psychological Support

1. Counseling and Therapy: Seeking help from a psychologist or counselor can provide emotional support. Cognitive-behavioral therapy (CBT) is particularly effective for managing stress and anxiety.

2. Support Groups: Joining a support group for cancer patients provides a sense of community and shared experience, which can be comforting.

3. Mindfulness and Meditation: Practices like

mindfulness meditation, progressive muscle relaxation, and guided imagery can reduce stress and improve overall well-being.

4. Journaling: Writing about feelings and experiences can be a therapeutic way to process emotions and reduce stress.

Conclusion

In conclusion, Lifestyle factors play a significant role in influencing the risk of developing cancer. Understanding and modifying these factors can lead to a substantial reduction in cancer risk.

lifestyle factors significantly influence cancer risk. Adopting a healthy diet, engaging in regular physical activity, maintaining a healthy weight, avoiding tobacco and excessive alcohol consumption, protecting against UV radiation, and minimizing exposure to environmental and occupational carcinogens are all effective strategies for reducing cancer risk.

Public health initiatives and personal lifestyle modifications, supported by ongoing research and education, can lead to substantial reductions in cancer incidence and improve overall health outcomes.

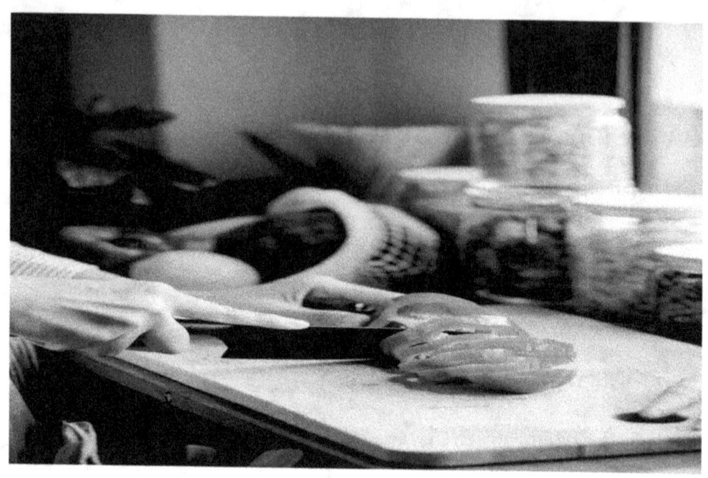

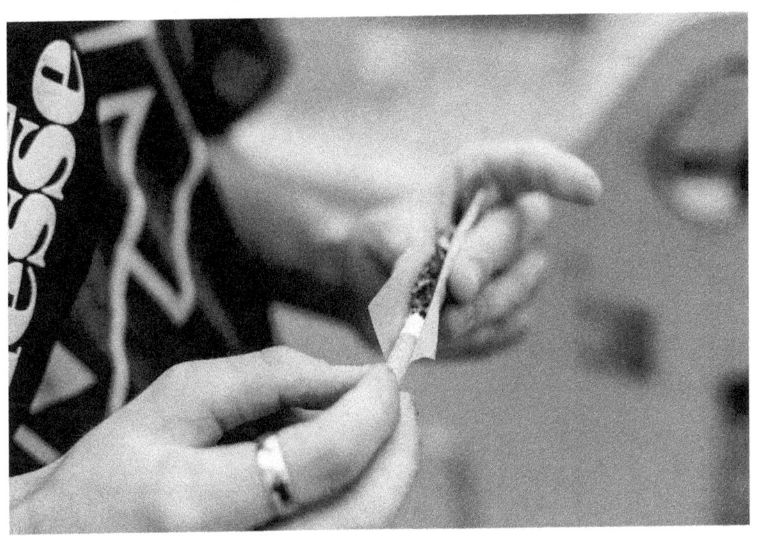